# YOUR KNOWLEDGE HAS VALUE

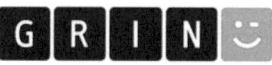
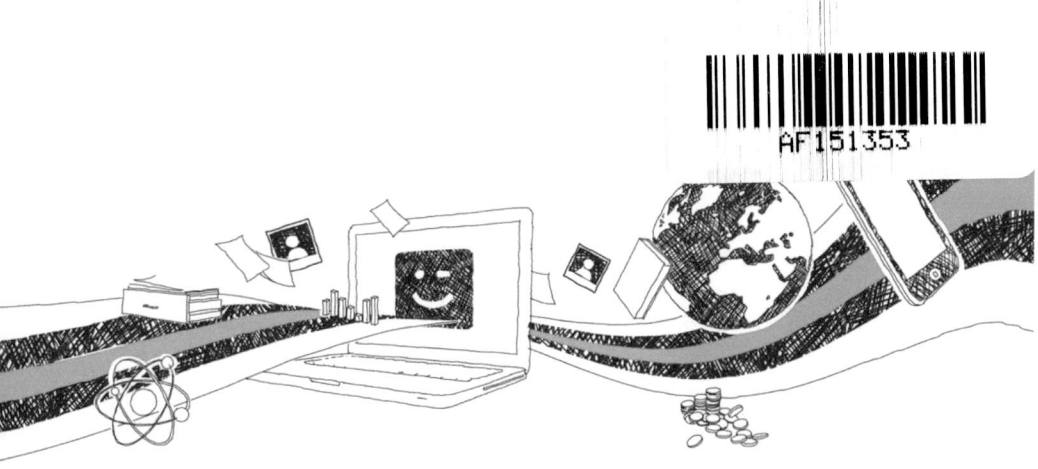

Ryan Borchers

# The Effects of Lysergic Acid Diethylamide

GRIN Publishing

**Bibliographic information published by the German National Library:**

The German National Library lists this publication in the National Bibliography; detailed bibliographic data are available on the Internet at http://dnb.dnb.de .

**Imprint:**

Copyright © 2014 GRIN Verlag GmbH
Print and binding: Books on Demand GmbH, Norderstedt Germany
ISBN: 978-3-656-86363-2

**This book at GRIN:**

http://www.grin.com/en/e-book/285595/the-effects-of-lysergic-acid-diethylamide

**GRIN - Your knowledge has value**

Since its foundation in 1998, GRIN has specialized in publishing academic texts by students, college teachers and other academics as e-book and printed book. The website www.grin.com is an ideal platform for presenting term papers, final papers, scientific essays, dissertations and specialist books.

**Visit us on the internet:**

http://www.grin.com/

http://www.facebook.com/grincom

http://www.twitter.com/grin_com

The Effects of Lysergic Acid Diethylamide

Ryan Borchers

The College of New Jersey

**Abstract**

The purpose of this research paper is to explain the history of Lysergic Acid Diethylamide (LSD) and the effects it has on the human body and brain. References to several studies are mentioned describing the effect LSD has on humans while under the influence of the drug, the effects LSD has on neurotransmitters in the brain, and the possible therapeutic benefits that can arise from proper treatment with the drug. The benefits and consequences that can occur from short and long term use are explained as well as possible side effects that can occur from using the drug. The connection between LSD and hallucinogen persisting perception disorder (HPPD) is explained and several myths focusing on the dangers and side effects of LSD are also debunked. It has been discovered that there are many positive benefits between LSD therapy and several diseases such as alcoholism, cluster headaches, and terminally ill patients.

Lysergic Acid Diethylamide, more commonly known as LSD, acid, L, or lucy, was first synthesized on November 16th, 1938 by Swiss chemist Albert Hofmann. It was not until April 19th, 1943 when Dr. Hofmann intentionally ingested some of his own LSD that the hallucinogenic properties were found. On that day, Hofmann ingested 250 micrograms of the substance which he predicted would be a threshold dose. He began to feel an intense sudden change in his perception and asked his lab assistant to help escort him home by bicycle. During the ride he claimed to feel intense waves of anxiety and was convinced that the LSD and poisoned him in some way. When he arrived home he contacted the doctor who arrived to his house only to determine that nothing seemed to be wrong with the exception of dilated pupils. After the doctor left, Hofmann started feeling better and bean to enjoy the closed eye visuals consisting of a wave of colors and geometric shapes that were influenced by the drug. He then realized he had discovered a very powerful psychoactive drug capable of producing a model psychosis. In the LSD community, this day is now known as Bicycle day in honor of Hofmann's discovery (Smith, 2014).

LSD is extremely potent, and its effects can be felt with as little as 20 micrograms of the substance. An average dose of LSD with noticeable hallucinogenic effects is anywhere between 100-200 micrograms. LSD can administered in a variety of ways including orally through blotters, liquid, sugar cubes, gelatin, or by pill. It is most commonly sold in blotters or 'tabs' which are small pieces of paper usually measuring 1cm by 1cm and often feature a design of some sort (Anderson, 1992). On the street, these blotters sell at an average of $10 each.

The effects are first noted about 20-40 minutes after ingestion with a sense of euphoria and light dizziness. The drug begins to reach its peak after an hour and plateau for about 4-5 hours before beginning to wear off after around 6-8 hours in. During the 'trip', users report feeling a separation of their ego, and ease of transition between states of consciousness. Many people also state that it sometimes difficult to fall asleep after the trip and that they usually have a decrease in appetite during it. A loss in perception is also common, which is what leads to the visual and auditory hallucinations felt by many people. Many users will report that they can see movement in static objections and will describe it as if a wall or ceiling was breathing or swirling. While under the influence of the drug, users usually have difficulty describing their experience through words and have trouble keeping track of thoughts or maintaining a conversation. 'Thought loops' occasionally occur while on higher doses in which a user will begin to think or talk about something, lose track of what they were thinking and begin to repeat or get stuck on the same thought. Many people report these thought loops as frightening and sometimes think that they are going insane. Occasionally people will report synesthesia while using the drug, which is when a sense is stimulated by a different sense, such as seeing music or hearing colors. The mood of the user can drastically change throughout the duration of the trip, people can often go from a relaxed euphoric state to a state of panic due to environmental conditions or internal thoughts. After a night of sleep the effects are almost always gone the next day (Anderson, 1992).

The long term effects of LSD can be both positive and negative. Many people report having their entire lives turned around for the better after using LSD. Other people have also gone to the hospital for 'LSD psychosis'. In a study done on analyzing these LSD psychosis patients, it was found that people who have a large family history of major psychosis or psychopathology and more vulnerable to experience LSD psychosis than those who do not (Tsuang et al., 1982). Some people also report suffering from 'LSD flashbacks' or HPPD which I will discuss further later in this paper. Winkler and Csémy (2014) conducted a study done amongst Czech Health Professionals who voluntarily partook in self-ingestion of LSD during its era of legal research between the years of 1952-1974. 22 health professionals, all either psychologists or psychiatrists, were interviewed on their long term effects of LSD usage. The interview consisted of 30 open-ended questions including where they underwent their experiment, the influence it had on them, their current opinion on LSD, and their reactions to a series of LSD related quotes read to them. All 22 of the participants claimed that they suffered no long term effects from LSD, and 20 of the 22 reported the experience to have a positive long-term effect on them in the area of either self-awareness or in the awareness in the world of a mentally ill patient. 19 of the 22 also reported that it allowed them to broaden their self-understanding and better understand the mind of the mentally ill.

There is limited research on how exactly LSD affects the brain. It is believed that LSD works similarly to serotonin. Serotonin is used in regulating appetite, sleep, mood, muscle control, sexuality and sensory perception. An experiment was done on rats to determine the relationship of the $5HT_{1A}$ receptor and LSD. Twelve rats were examined over a period of six weeks and given LSD of varying amounts. The $5HT_{1A}$ receptor showed increased stimulation during the tests which supports the theory that $5HT_{1A}$ plays a significant role while under the influence of LSD (Reissig, Eckler, Rabin, & Winter, 2005). LSD also plays a role in the change of regulation of many other neurotransmitters and receptors, including dopamine, adrenal receptors and the release of glutamate in the cerebral cortex (Evans, 2013). After ingestion, a person will develop a rapid tolerance build up to most hallucinogens that effect similar receptors. This tolerance will last a couple days while the neurotransmitters are restored back to their optimal levels. The research available on LSD has been very limited for the past few decades which is preventing us from understanding exactly how this drug affects the brain.

The effects of LSD have been experimented with by governments for many years during the 1950's and 1960's. Its initial research with the CIA and military was to determine if the effects could be manipulated to create a psychological weapon and act as a 'mind control' drug or truth serum. After these tests failed, the government outlawed LSD in 1966 and later classified it as a .Schedule 1 drug under the Controlled Substances Act in 1970. After this classification, all therapeutic trials came to a halt, and research was stopped for many years. It was not until this past decade that research was again permitted on the therapeutic potential of LSD and other hallucinogenic drugs (Smith, Raswyck & Dickerson, 2014).

Before its outlaw, LSD was tested with a number of therapeutic techniques in order to try and determine its positive therapeutic benefits. As I stated earlier in this paper, LSD can provide a large increase in self-understanding. Someone dealing with depression or an addiction may be able to face the reality of their situation and begin the process of recovery. Krebs and Johansen (2012) conducted an experiment on the effects of treating alcoholism with LSD. They performed their experiment over the course of six studies with 536 participants. Three hundred twenty-five of these participants had been randomly assigned to receive a full dose of LSD and the other 211 were assigned to the control group. These participants were assigned a varying dose of LSD depending on the study. One hundred eighty-five of the 315 patients (59%) and only 73 of the 191 control patients (38%) had indicated they had abstained from drinking at the first three-month follow up after receiving one dose of LSD. The patients unaccounted for had chosen to drop out of the study.

An amazing discovery was found that shows great potential in the usage of LSD and psilocybin in the alleviation of cluster headaches. Cluster headaches are described as one of the most painful experiences can have. They involve an intense, unbearable pain, usually on one side of the face which can last up to 90 minutes and occur several times a day. Those who suffer from cluster headaches usually develop them in periods that can last many weeks. Sewell, Halpern and Pope Jr. (2006) interviewed 53 cluster headache patients, all of who had either tried using psilocybin or LSD in order to treat their condition. 25 out of 48 (52%) participants who have claimed to use psilocybin and 7 out of 8 (88%) participants who claimed to use LSD to treat their condition state that their cluster headaches were no longer occurring during their usual cluster headache periods. I find this study to be fascinating considering there are no known medications able to treat cluster headaches, but these drugs can offer a source of temporary relief.

Templer, Arikawa, and Gariety (2004) reviewed studies done with psychopathic drugs on terminally ill patients. One of these studies involved the use of LSD on terminally ill patients in an effort to reduce anxiety and help provide a sense of peace and acceptance with their remaining time. The study consisted of 22 terminal cancer patients who had been treated with LSD in order to achieve six main components. "(1) sense of unity and oneness (positive ego transcendence and loss of usual sense of self without loss of consciousness), (2) transcendence of time and space, (3) deeply felt positive mood (joy, peace and love), (4) sense of awareness and reverence, (5) meaningfulness of psychological and/or philosophical insight, and (6) ineffability (sense of difficulty in communicating the experience by verbal description)." Each patient had one session lasting 10-14 hours assisted with family photographs and music. Afterwards the patients spent time with their families in order to evaluate the effectiveness of the treatment. 14 out of 22 patients showed improvement and a permanent reduced level of anxiety.

A rare effect from LSD usage is Hallucinogen persisting perception disorder (HPPD). The DSM-IV defines HPPD as "The re-experiencing, following cessation of use of a hallucinogen, of one or more of the perceptual symptoms that were experienced while intoxicated with the hallucinogen (e.g., geometric hallucinations, false perceptions of movement in the peripheral visual fields, flashes of colors, intensified colors, trails of images of moving objects, positive afterimages, halos around objects, micropsia, and macropsia." (American Psychiatric Association, 2000). Not much information is known about the true cause of HPPD. It has been predicted that it might be caused by the destruction of inhibitory neurons which are responsible for regulating and filtering sensory information. It has also been predicted that it's caused by dis-inhibition of the Catechol-$O$-methyltransferase (COMT) enzyme which is responsible for the breakdown of catecholamines in the brain. This would prevent sensory gating, which is the filtering of unnecessary stimuli by the brain and would explain the effects of HPPD. Many people who claim to have HPPD will experience it early on with their hallucinogen usage and sometimes even after their first try. Many other people who have used hallucinogens hundreds of times report never getting it (Subramanian, & Doran, 2014). Due to this interesting nature of the disorder, it is possible that those who develop HPPD might have due to an underlying hereditary factor. There are no medications that are able to cure HPPD. Many doctors will often prescribe a benzodiazepine such as Clonazepam to help treat the disorder, but they are often ineffective.

LSD often receives a negative view by most Americans and especially by our government. There are dozens of myths and propaganda that people hear about LSD which only fuels their misconception about the drug. LSD is not an addictive substance, nor are most hallucinogens. There is a common myth that LSD will stay in the body or spinal fluid forever. Studies done in the 1960's have debunked this myth and confirmed that LSD has a half-life of 175 minutes which would mean that LSD is virtually out of the body in one day. LSD is also almost impossible to overdose on. The LD-50 of LSD in humans is predicted to range between 0.2mg/kg to 1mg/kg. This absurd amount would be thousands times more than the recreational average dose. The only reported overdose was a 34 year old man who had injected 320mg (160,000-320,000 times the average dose) of LSD intravenously (Griggs & Ward, 1977).

We have slowly begun to reverse the steps taken decades before and have allowed LSD to be researched again. LSD does not have the reputation it once had with only being associated with hippies and drug addicts. The National Institute of Drug Abuse (NIDA) reports that over 34 million (11.0%) Americans age 26 and older have tried LSD at least once in their lives (NIDA, 2013). In the short history we have with this drug, there have already been discoveries that can help treat many conditions and disorders ranging from alcoholism to cluster headaches. With over 40 years of potential research gone, there are countless studies to be conducted with our new technology that can help us better determine the therapeutic benefits and long term effects of LSD usage.

References

American Psychiatric Association. (2000). *Diagnostic and statistical manual of mental disorders*

(4th ed., text rev.). doi:10.1176/appi.books.9780890423349.

Anderson, M. (1992, July 28). The Psychological Effects of LSD. Retrieved from

https://www.erowid.org/chemicals/lsd/lsd_effects1.shtml

Dyck, E. (2005). Flashback: Psychiatric Experimentation With LSD in Historical Perspective.

*The Canadian Journal of Psychiatry / La Revue Canadienne De Psychiatrie, 50*(7), 381-

388.                           Retrieved                           from

http://eds.a.ebscohost.com/ehost/pdfviewer/pdfviewer?sid=e19a3e6b-8a6a-4b11-84a4-

29026d94bea3%40sessionmgr4005&vid=10&hid=4103

Evans, B. (2013, November 5). LSD Effects on the Brain - The Human Brain Project. Retrieved

from http://www.thehumanbrainproject.org/lsd-effects-brain/

Griggs, E. A., & Ward, M. (1977, May 25). LSD toxicity: a suspected cause of death. *J Ky Med*

*Association,*                    75(4):172-3.                    Retrieved                    from

https://www.erowid.org/chemicals/lsd/lsd_death.shtml

Krebs, T. S., & Johansen, P. (2012). Lysergic acid diethylamide (LSD) for alcoholism: Meta-

analysis of randomized controlled trials. *Journal of Psychopharmacology, 26*(7), 994-

1002. doi:10.1177/0269881112439253

Lev-Ran, S., Feingold, D., Frenkel, A., & Lerner, A. G. (2014). Clinical characteristics of

individuals with schizophrenia and hallucinogen persisting perception disorder: A

preliminary    investigation.    *Journal    of    Dual    Diagnosis,    10*(2),    79-83.

doi:10.1080/15504263.2014.906155

Lyvers, M., & Meester, M. (2012). Illicit use of LSD or psilocybin, but not MDMA or nonpsychedelic drugs, is associated with mystical experiences in a dose-dependent manner. *Journal of Psychoactive Drugs, 44*(5), 410-417. doi:10.1080/02791072.2012.736842

National Institute of Drug Abuse. (2013). Hallucinogens. Retrieved from http://www.drugabuse.gov/drugs-abuse/hallucinogens

Reissig, C. J., Eckler, J. R., Rabin, R. A., & Winter, J. C. (2005). The 5-HT1A receptor and the stimulus effects of LSD in the rat. *Psychopharmacology, 182*(2), 197-204. doi:10.1007/s00213-005-0068-6

Smith, D. E., Raswyck, G. E., & Dickerson-Davidson, L. (2014). From Hofmann to the Haight Ashbury, and into the future: The past and potential of lysergic acid diethlyamide. *Journal of Psychoactive Drugs, 46*(1), 3-10. doi:10.1080/02791072.2014.873684

Subramanian, N. N., & Doran, M. M. (2014). Improvement of hallucinogen persisting perception disorder (HPPD) with oral risperidone: Case report. *Irish Journal of Psychological Medicine, 31*(1), 47-49. doi:10.1017/ipm.2013.59

Winkler, P., & Csémy, L. (2014). Self-experimentations with psychedelics among mental health professionals: LSD in the former Czechoslovakia. *Journal of Psychoactive Drugs, 46*(1), 11-19. doi:10.1080/02791072.2013.873158